Joanfielding@comcast.net

Story and Graphics by

Joan Fielding

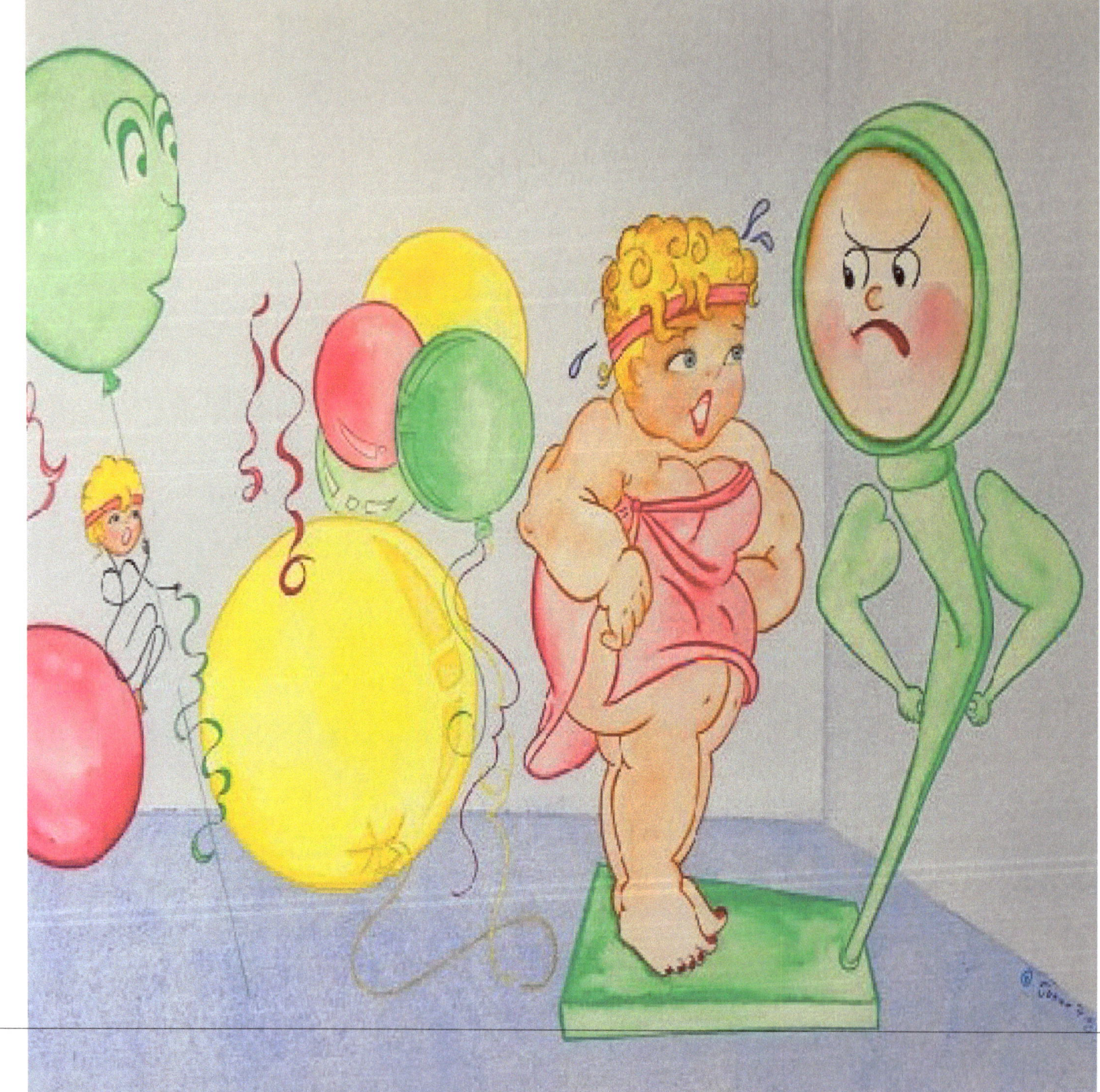

Weigh In And Begin
Your New Year Right.
Your Goal: To Be Thin
One Year From Tonight.

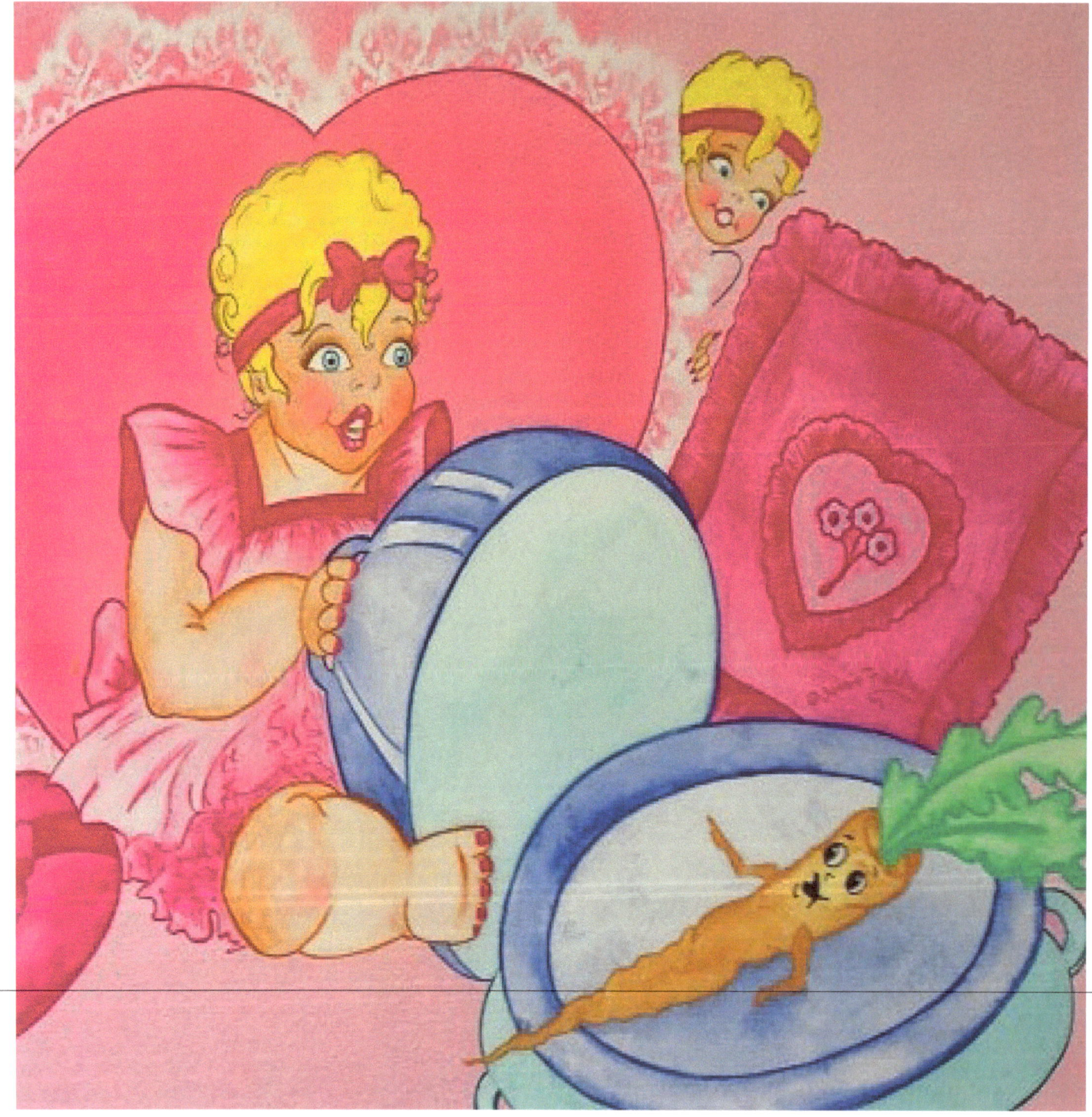

Stick To The Carrot Sticks
And You Will See,
Someone's Valentine
You Will Surely Be.

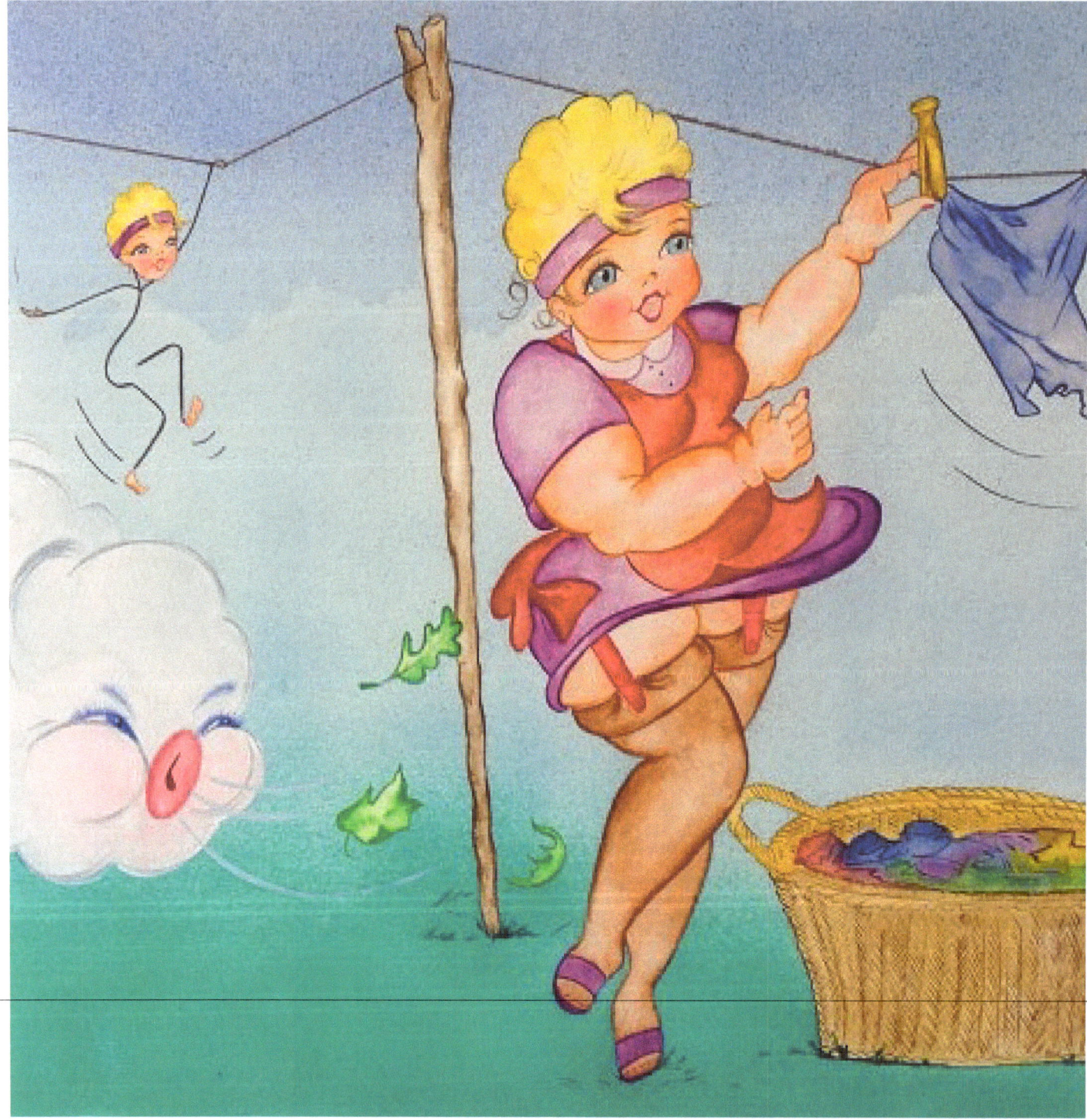

The Winds of March
May Blow and Blow,
You're Losing Weight
It's Starting To Show.

_____

_____

_____

_____

_____

_____

_____

_____

_____

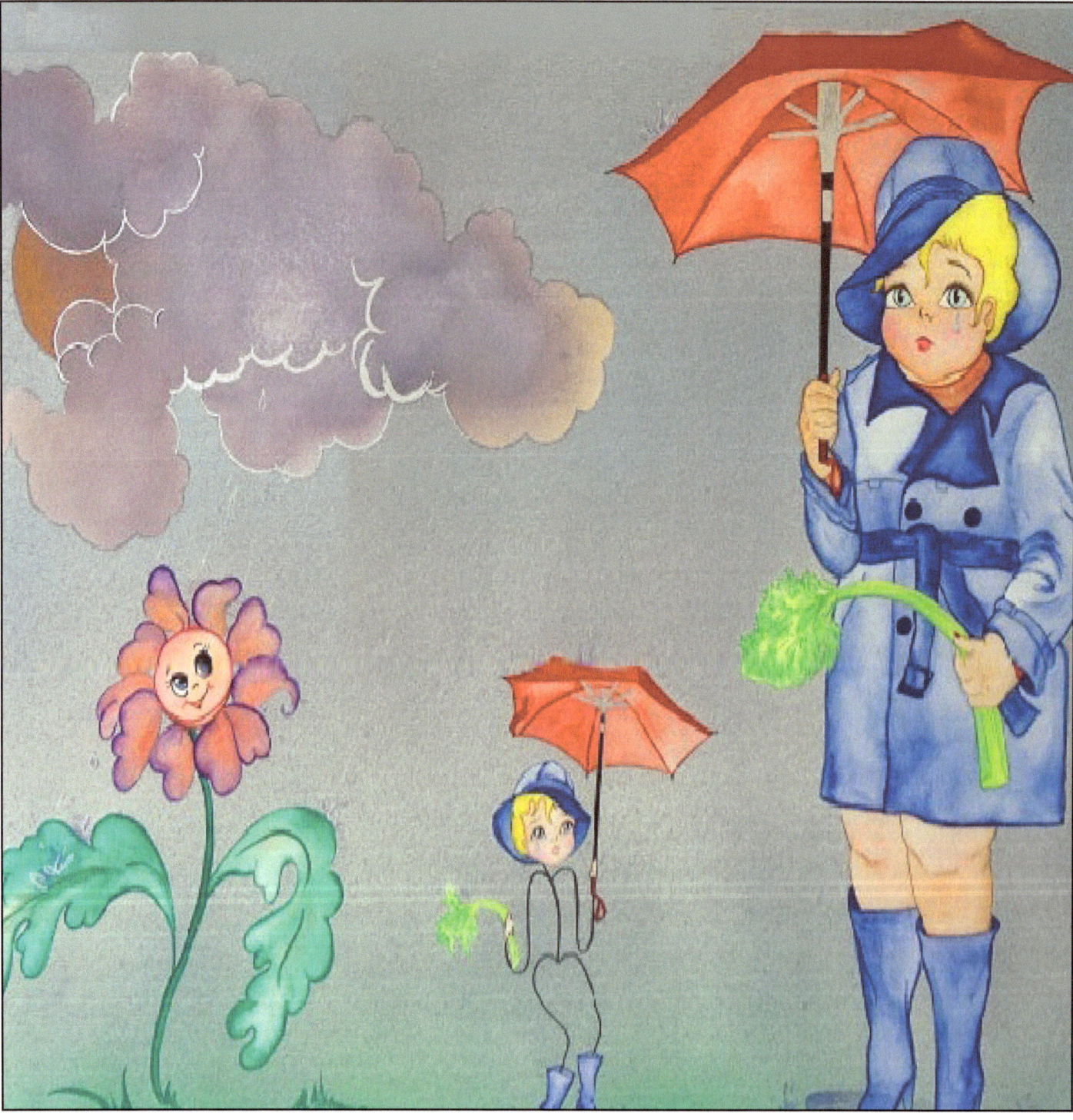

April Showers
Bring May Flowers.
Pounds Come Off With
Sheer Will Power.

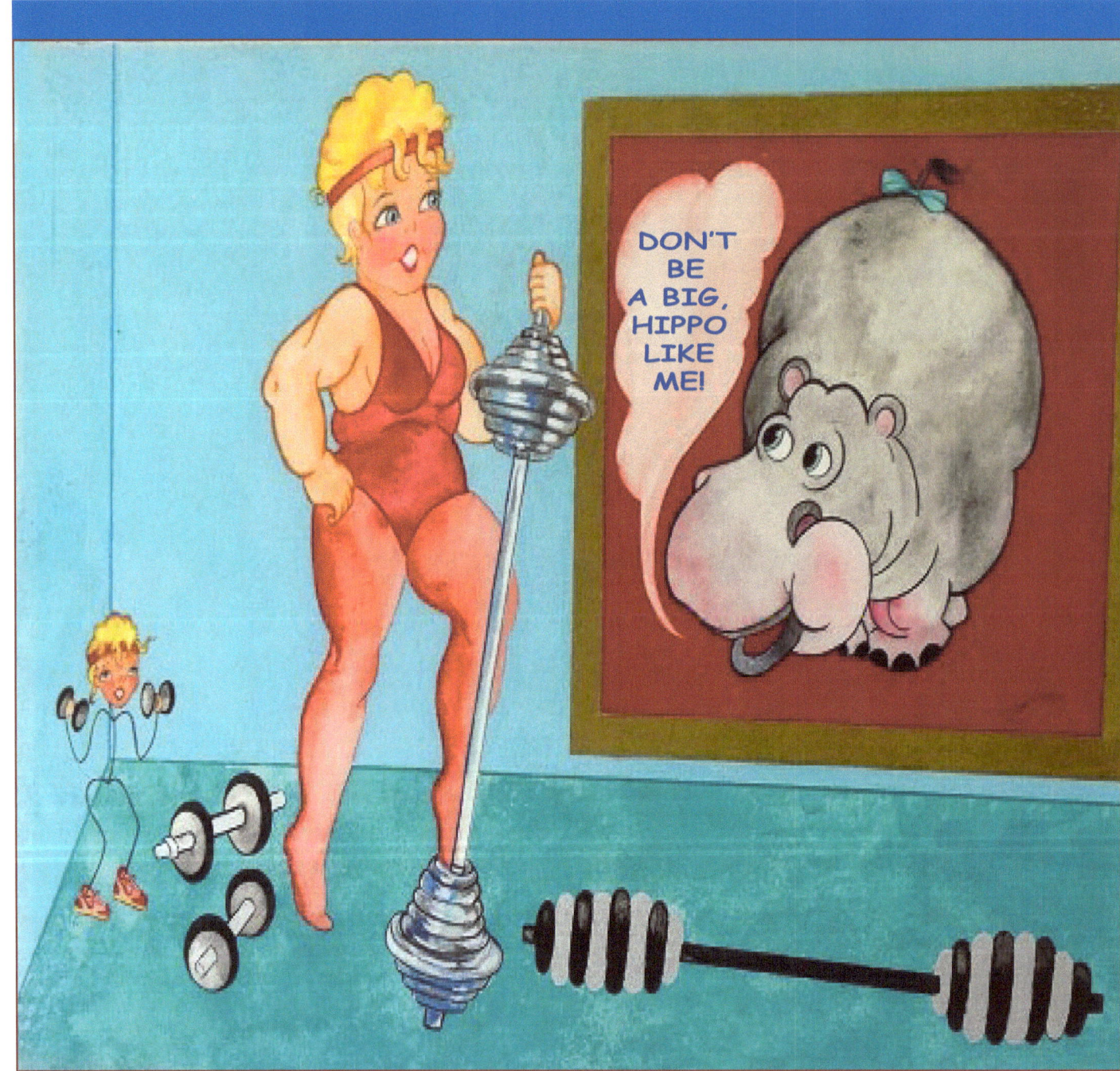

Memorial Day Will
Find You Strong When
You Think Of All
The Pounds That Are Gone.

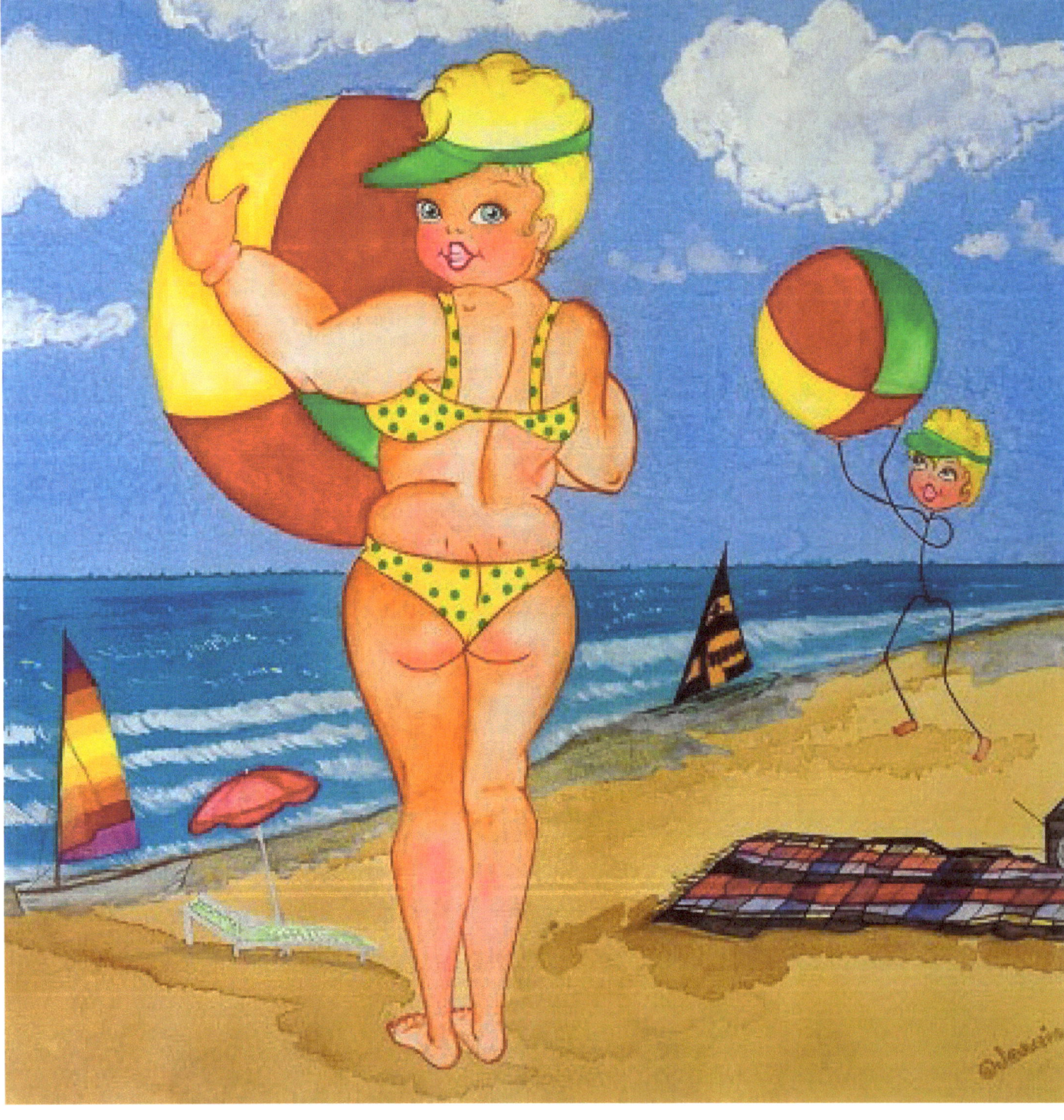

Time For The Beach
And Don't You Look Cute
In Your New
Bikini Bathing Suit.

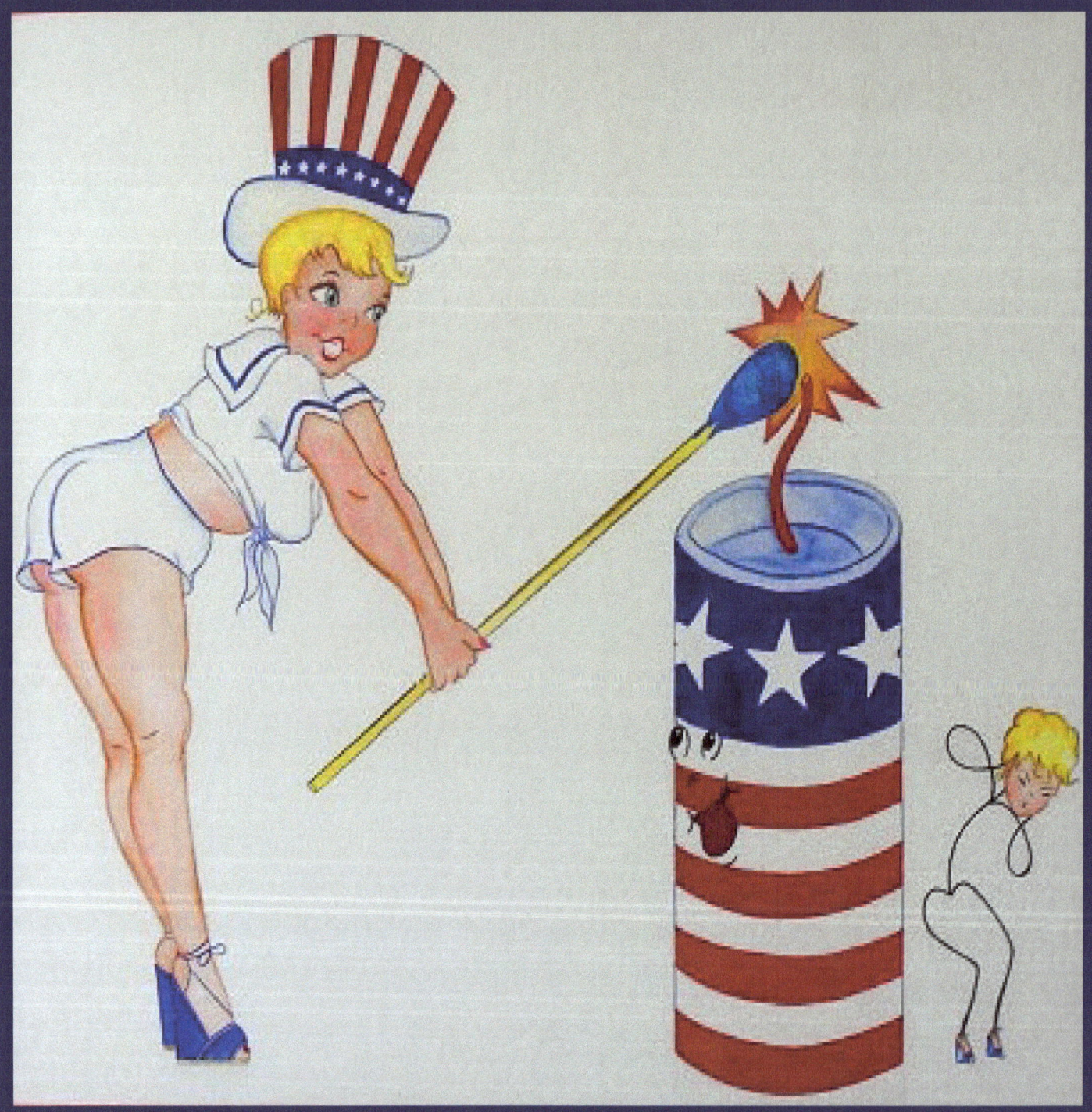

The 4th Of July,
The Red, White And Blue.
A Firecracker Day--
And You're One Too!

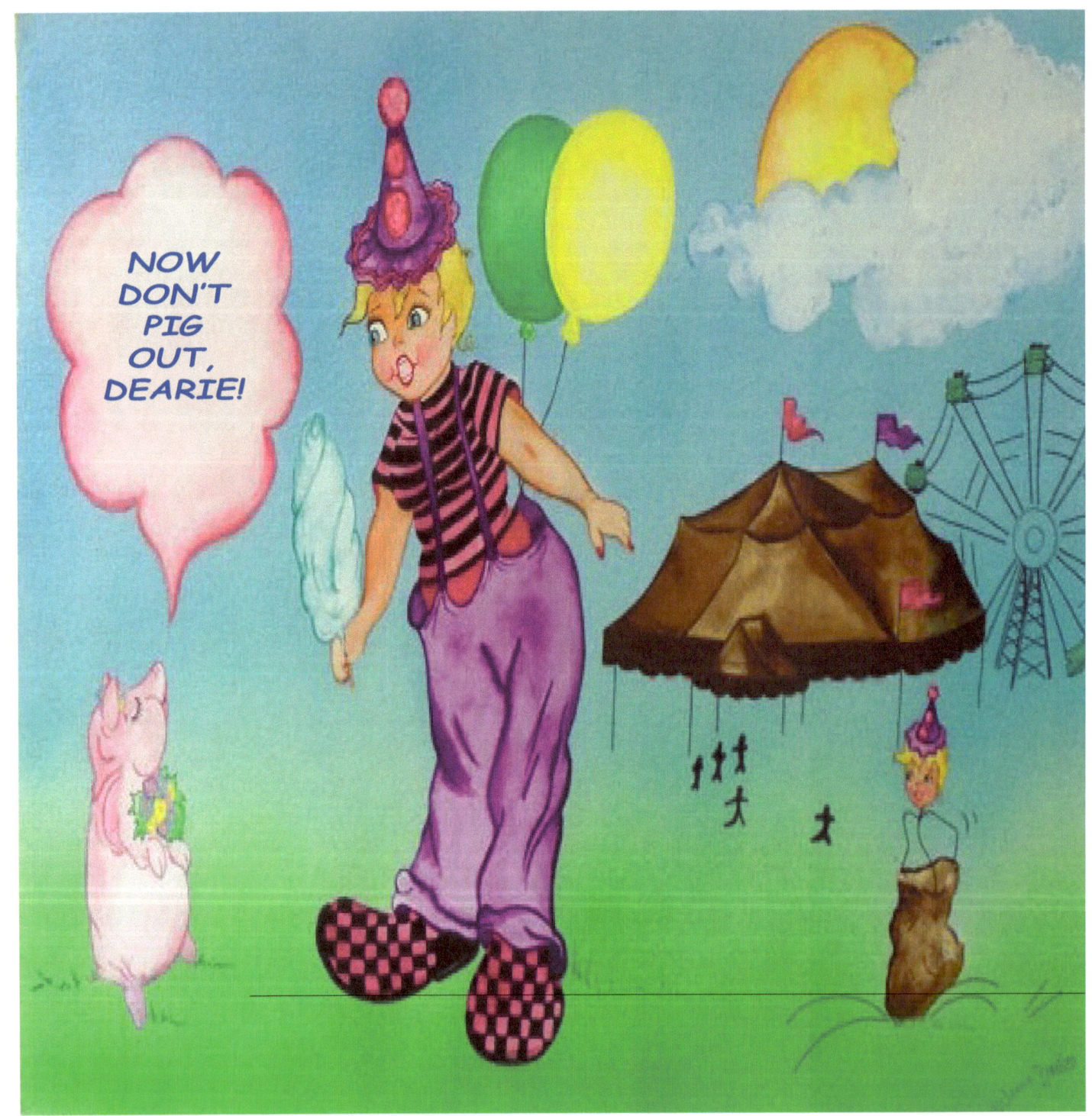

August Is Here; The Deadline Draws Near. Only Four Months To Go You'll Make It My Dear.

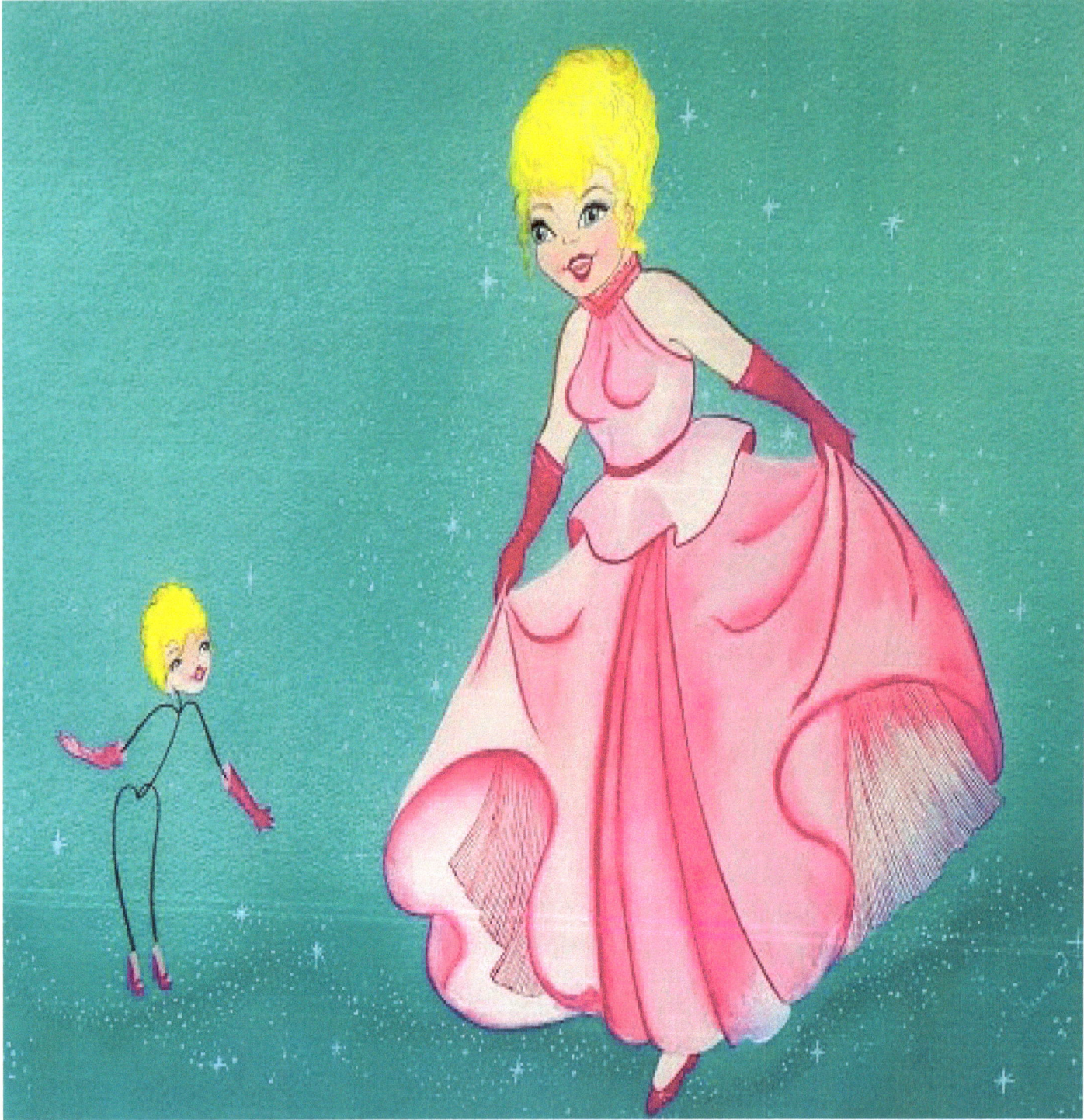

You Earned A Reward
For Being So Good.
You Stuck To Your Diet
Like A Good Girl Should.

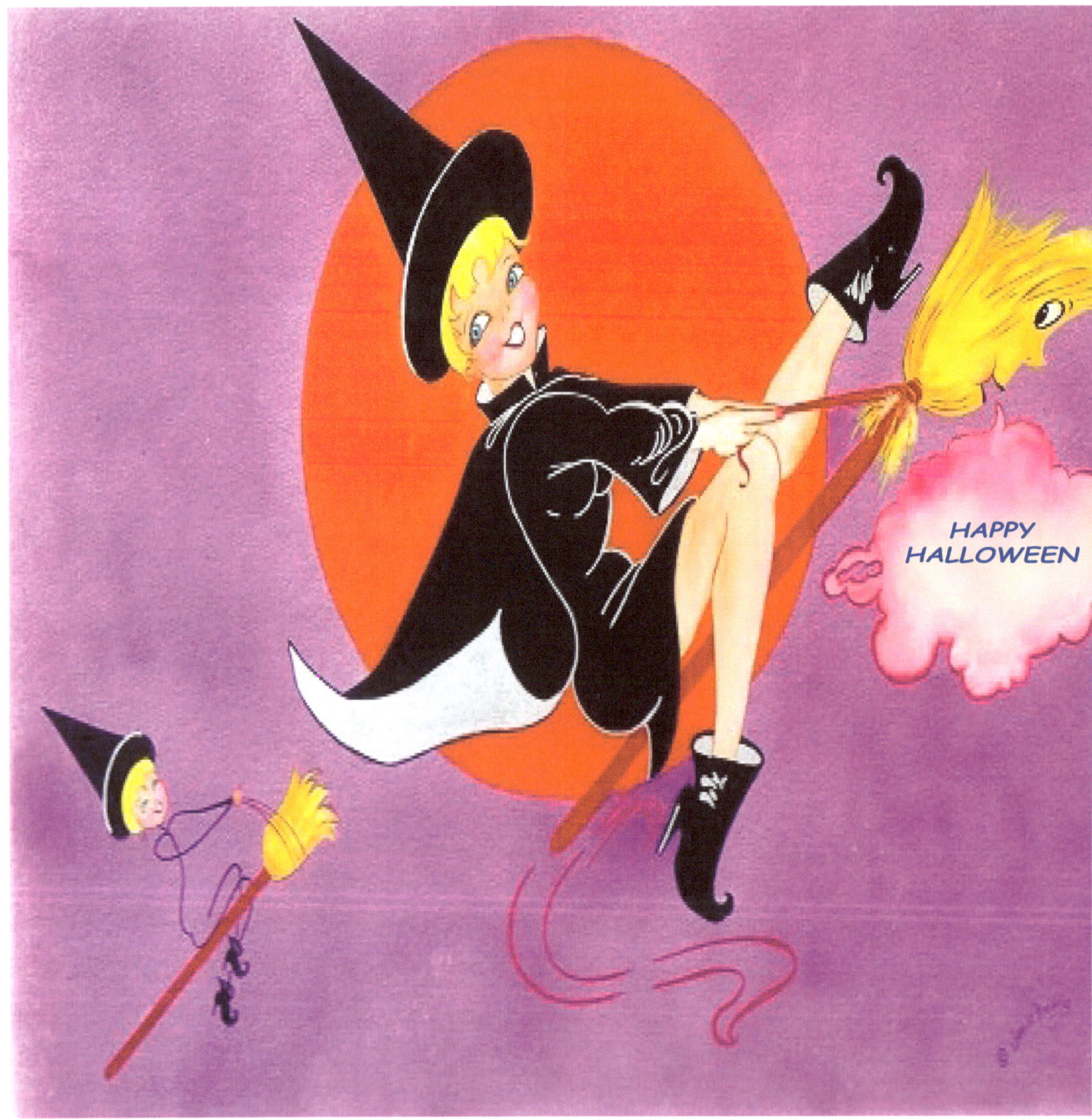

This Is The Month For
Trick And Treating. Do
All Of The Tricks
Not All Of The Eating.

_____

_____

_____

_____

_____

_____

_____

_____

_____

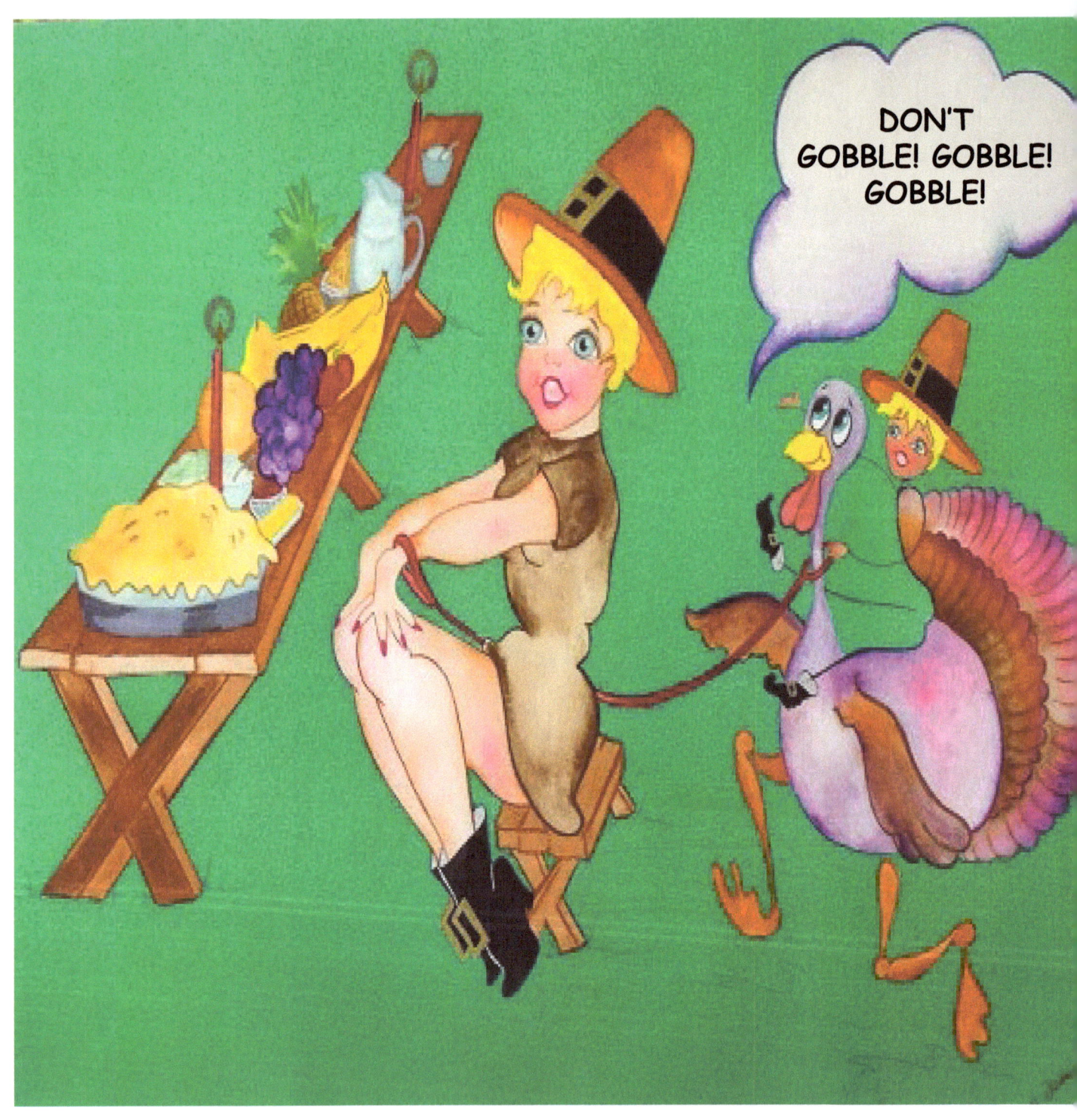

Time For Turkey
Minced Pie And Such.
Look At The Goodies--
But Don't Eat Too Much.

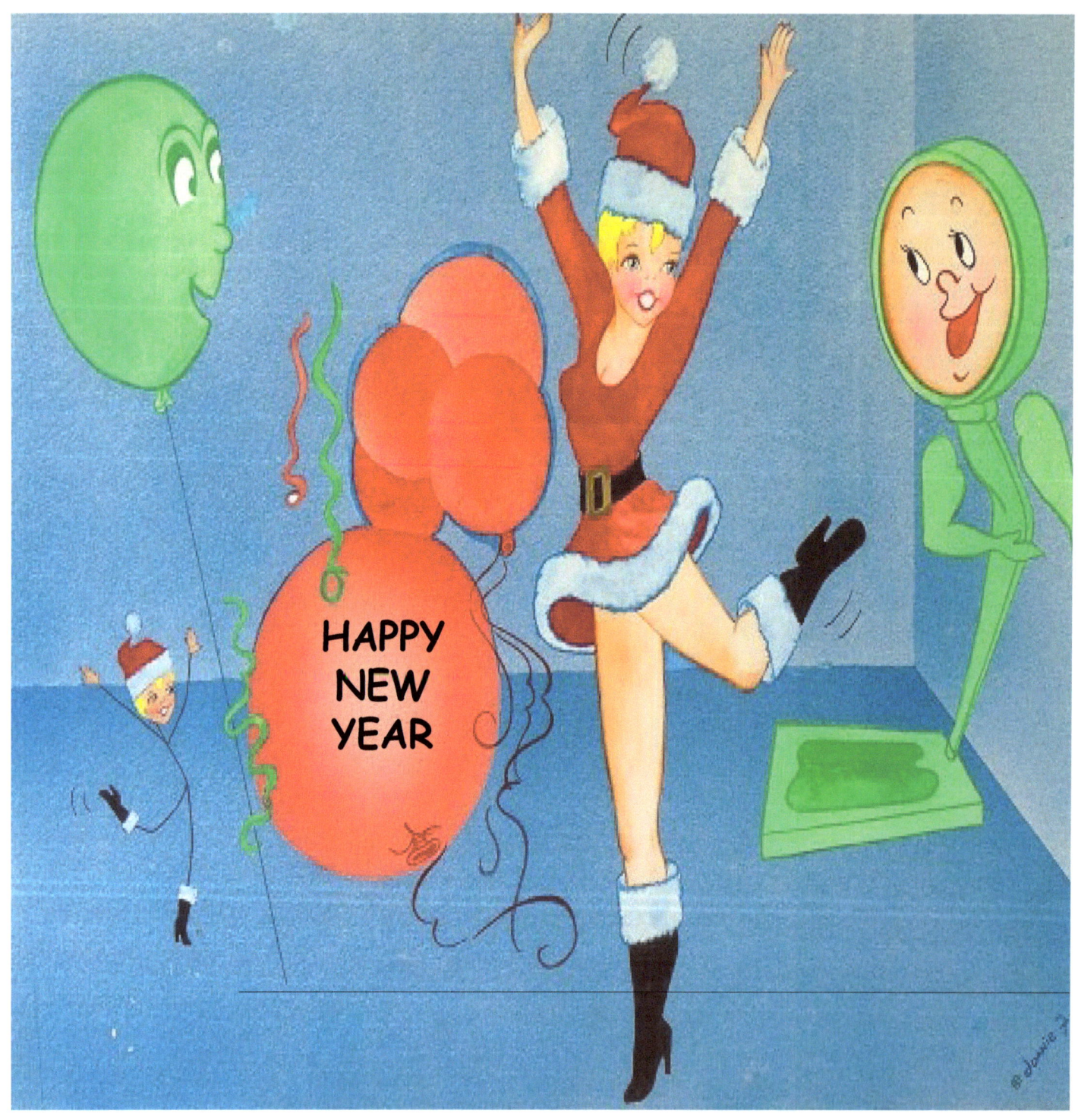

A New Year Begins,
The Scale Says Your Thin.
Winners Never Quit,
Quitters Never Win.

_____

_____

_____

_____

_____

_____

_____

_____

_____

_____